Contents

Natural Weight Loss:

PROVEN Strategies for Healthy Weight Loss & Accelerated Metabolism

By C.K. Murray

Weight loss doesn't have to be hard.

If you're struggling day after day to shed those pesky pounds—and *keep* them off—it's time to rethink your approach. Not only is weight loss possible, but it is highly *probable*, if you do the right things. Shrinking your waistline is about more than simply burning fat. It's about living healthier, and taking those small, easy steps that make your dream body a reality. Build lean muscle, boost metabolic rates, and turn *today's* body into *tomorrow's* fine-tuned, calorie-burning furnace.

No joke. All science.

So stop looking in the mirror and feeling bad. Stop stepping on the scale and losing hope. If you don't like the person you're becoming, know that you have the power to change. While it is true that we are all born with different body chemistries, and that our environments constantly play a role, we also *all* possess the power to transform.

If you're seeking a natural means to losing weight, one independent of risky dieting pills, experimental drugs, invasive surgeries, and unhealthy diet fads, you've come to the right place. In the following pages you will learn how to shed pounds and gain energy, all the while improving your health in the <u>long-term</u>. These strategies are designed to ensure weight loss that endures for the rest of your life.

If you're seeking unnatural and immediate weight loss, this book is not for you. However, if you want to lose weight in a way that is healthy and sustainable, in a manner that strengthens your body and your mind, then continue reading.

But enough is enough. Let's quit the pep talk and get right down to the facts…

Where Do YOU Weigh In?

Are you *obese* or *overweight*?

Perhaps you don't want to think about it, but there *is* a difference. We all approach this life with different backgrounds and motivations. Some people can eat like crap their entire lives and maintain great physiques. Others can work their tails off only to remain heavy.

In the end, what matters is consistency. If you can become consistent in your habits, your thoughts, your behaviors, then you can and *will* lose weight.

And if you're losing the will to keep going, know that you are not alone. In fact, the World Health Organization (WHO) estimates that over 1.4 billion adults were overweight in 2008, with over 200 million men and 300 million women being obese. When it comes to distinguishing between overweight and obese, the WHO defines *overweight* as a Body mass index (BMI) of 25 or over, and *obese* as a BMI of 30 or more.

If you're wondering how a BMI is calculated, it's a basic formula. Simply take your weight in kilograms divided by the square of your height in meters (kg/m^2). Still, if all this seems a little funky and you're not interested in calculating your BMI, know this: *your life could depend on it.*

Around 3.4 million adults die each year because of obesity or overweightness. 44% of diabetes and 41% of cancers are attributable to being overweight and obese. So if any of this is making you scared or killing your motivation, think otherwise!

Let your fear be your motivation! Allow your need for change guide you to that change.

Let's do this!

Brain Fat -- The Weight Loss Power of Neurogenic Visualization

At this point, you're probably scratching your head. "What in the heck is *neurogenic visualization?*"

Well, let's start with the basics. You see, visualization is an active, open focus on a goal or image. It is practiced and preached in sports across the world, used as a guide to artistic achievement, and implemented in Fortune 500 companies as part of a powerful yet simple motivational strategy.

Basically, visualization is not a bunch of nonsense. It has very real and far-reaching implications, and has been the cornerstone of long-lasting spiritual practices across time and culture. And the reason is simple.

Weight loss doesn't start in the belly or intestine. It doesn't have origins in our fat cells nor in our digestive tract, nor somewhere in the foods we ingest.

Weight loss, and weight gain, start in the brain.

Ask any serious athlete about his or her sport. Question an artist on the intricacies of the craft. Chances are, that person will tell you that preparation begins well before the perfect game or masterpiece occurs. And it's not just about the hours, days, months, and years of practicing.

It's not just the physical act of doing.

Much of what brings success to people in these careers, and in many other walks of life, is the power of visualization. The ability to align oneself with a clear and realistic image of success.

A baseball player imagines himself at the plate, taking balls and forcing the pitcher to throw that perfect hittable strike-zone pitch. A soccer player visualizes moving down the field, weaving through defenders, seamlessly and confidently making way to the goal for that clutch kick. A painter visualizes the contour of that next artistic image; a writer visualizes the world of the character, the way that world looks and feels and tastes—and how that character's thoughts and behaviors filter through.

It doesn't matter what your goal is. If you're at the bottom rung of a company, you can visualize yourself going through every day, doing your best, impressing your bosses, your coworkers, and dominating your workload as you surely scale the corporate ladder. Visualization will work for the budding professional just as it will work for the kid on the basketball court trying to improve his jump shot. It will work for the avid bodybuilder trying to attain a hulking physique, just as it will work for the average Joe trying to shed a few pounds.

Visualization is the stepping stone for everything else—and in many ways, the most underrated action a person can take. Fortunately, none of the stigma or doubt surrounding visualization matters. That is, it doesn't matter, so long as you work it. And visualization *does* work.

But why? And how?

Before you become too skeptical, consider the case of a person with Body Dysmorphic Disorder (BDD). For those with this disorder, the smallest perceived physical flaw becomes a life-changer. Every day, the individual will feel terrible about the slightest thing—a crooked nose, small hands, the space between the eyes, pointy ears, lips that are too large or small, etc. In many cases, the perceived physical flaw is so negligible that others don't even notice it. However, for the individual with BDD, this flaw is the biggest problem in their world.

In short, individuals suffering from BDD visualize themselves as ugly and hideous. Their power of visualization (although negative) is so strong that it completely distorts their image. And this is not that uncommon. Consider anorexia and bulimia. These people think that they are fat when they are not. They look in the mirror and see a person who is overweight. They will look at others who are much heavier and will think these people look good, and then will continue to starve or purge in order to approach how they visualize these other, more 'beautiful' people.

On the other end, there are certain people who will look in the mirror and think that they are too skinny or bony, forcing themselves to eat more and more, even to the point of sickness. Regardless of the extremity, whether seeing ourselves as too fat or too skinny—it all begins in the brain.

The brain is a powerful thing, but we can change it. If we can learn to visualize a different image, a different outcome, a different ideal, then we can gradually, but surely, approach that new life.

Visualization physically changes the neural pathways in our brains. It creates a new perception of ourselves, our worlds, and those around us. So before you 'force' yourself to adopt the latest fad diet, or some strict regimen, think about your approach.

Remember that meditation and visualization have gone hand in hand for centuries. They form the beginning of human expansion, channeling the mind and body in a way that is as mystical as it is powerful. And boy oh boy is it powerful.

Visualization has been shown to:

Regulate the Nervous System

Balance Hormones

Improve Cognitive Performance

Improve Athletic Performance

Accelerate Metabolism

Lower Pulse

Lower Blood Pressure

Ward off Degenerative Diseases

When beginning to visualize, be honest with yourself. Weight gain is often the result of many factors. We can put on pounds due to stress, lack of sleep, hormonal imbalances, excessive eating, lack of exercise, maladaptive mindsets, and many other intersecting forces.

For some people, weight gain is the result of actually perceiving the need for a buffer. Subconsciously or consciously, their extra weight serves as a protective layer. They turn to food for safety. They eat not only because eating makes them feel good, but because it gives their body a physical plumpness that literally, and figuratively, cushions them against real-world stressors. As a result, their metabolism continues to slow and their eating continues.

Some people may not even eat unhealthily, but they continue to depend upon that 'buffer' for protection. They are afraid of shedding their shell, so to speak, and so their brain actually communicates to the body to hold on to weight. It is a defense mechanism, one that can become so engrained, that people rarely take the time to acknowledge it.

If all of this sounds like a bunch of nonsense, consider the science:

Obese people actually show premature aging in the white matter of their brains. This is related to what scientists call neurogenesis, or the growth of new neurons. Basically, our brains are *always* growing new neurons, a fact that opposes the long-standing belief that our brains become stale and fully grown early in our 20s.

One of the greatest areas of neurogenesis in our brains is the hypothalamus, which among other critical functions, deals directly with metabolism, hunger and thirst. Scientists have conducted studies on rats showing that neurogenesis changes in the brain, depending upon the diet fed. Rats fed high-fat diets begin to show a significant increase in neurogenesis. But instead of promoting learning or memory, these new neurons actually cause the rats to gain weight. In rats not fed high-fat diets, there is little to no neurogenesis of this type.

But this is where it gets _really_ interesting. In several studies, the scientists knew that the new neurons in the hypothalamus were associated with weight gain, but this was not enough.

So they killed them. They x-rayed and eradicated all the new neurons in the rats fed high-fat diets. They then continued to feed these rats the same high-fat diet, but with incredible results. These new rats, with the neurogenesis removed, showed little to no weight gain. Meanwhile, the other rats whose neurons were still intact continued to eat the high-fat diet and continued to gain significant weight and fat mass.

Most surprising of all, perhaps, was the fact that the rats with their neurons removed—despite eating high-fat diets—exhibited less weight gain than the more active rats.

Basically, the study confirmed one thing: weight gain is quite literally in the brain.

Scientists conjecture that humans are no different in this regard, as we all evolved to learn to eat as much as we could when it was available. This neurogenesis ensured that our hunter-gathering ancestors would eat whenever they came upon food. In the hunter-gatherer days we would have utilized all that high-fat for energy. It would have served us to collect vegetables and hunt large prey over long distances. However, in our modern day of supermarkets and restaurants and mass production, this evolutionary mechanism is no longer an advantage. The evolution of technology has outpaced the evolution of our brains.

In other words, our brain continues to tell us to eat, eat, eat the high-fat diet, even when it's actually hurting us.

Scientists have also discovered evolutionary mechanisms in another part our brains: the hippocampus. The hippocampus is a region closely tied to memory and learning, a region that is a wellspring of neurogenesis. Throughout our lives, the more we learn, the more neurons there are springing up in this area. No matter what we do—whether it's playing a sport, watching T.V., going to work, or making that morning cup of coffee—it all gets reinforced by our neurons. The more we do something, the more our neurons change to accommodate that behavior, and the more habitual that behavior becomes.

This is the basis of addiction. Drug addicts have such a hard time quitting their habit because their brains are literally wired differently than everybody else's. In many cases, the brain of the drug addict *stops* making other neurons to ensure that the neurons associated with drug use are in full supply.

Think of visualization the same way. The more you visualize a certain behavior and outcome, the more your neurons 'learn' the associated actions needed to reach that goal. Your hippocampus wires itself so that memories of visualized activities are engrained. Then, once your hippocampus has adequately created its supply of neurons, your hypothalamus (the area associated with metabolism, hunger and thirst) can further engrain these learned behaviors through its own neurogenesis.

Remember, all areas of our brain are linked. Although people may say that they're "right-brained" or "left-brained," there is really no such thing. A normal, healthy brain utilizes all areas. They are all interlinked. Yes, some people may have an aptitude for certain functions associated with one side over the other, but even so, *all* parts of the brain are used to an extent.

Now, reconsider the role of visualization in the brain. Part of being able to visualize is being able to enter a quasi-meditative state. What this means is that you enter a state of utmost relaxation. Before you can truly visualize, you need to clear your head. You need to stop thinking about your errands, your insecurities, your friends and family, your past regrets and future worries.

Before you can visualize, you need to create the mental space for imagery. So clear your mind of the clutter. Make that space a blank slate, and allow the desire images to construct before your closed eyes. And by all means, understand that what you are doing is more than simply daydreaming.

Meditative states have a very real impact on the brain. In fact, research now shows that Meditation is like a gym workout for your brain. The latest neuroimaging supports this. Areas of our noggin for attention, learning and emotional regulation will actually change in shape and size with meditation and visualization. Neuroimaging now reveals significant improvements in grey matter density and thickness in the brain.

In fact, meditators and visualizers show the same level of thickness as nonmeditators 20 years younger, despite assertions that thickness decreases with age. This goes against everything that scientists have been claiming for a long time. Basically, meditation and visualization strengthen the frontal cortex and insula, improving the capacity for decision-making, planning, and judgment. Not to mention, memory, emotional balance, and the ability to multitask.

In other words, the evidence is telling. If you want to lose weight, you need to visualize what you want to do. Before you begin some new diet regimen, before you dive full-on into some drastic measure to shred weight, visualize the process.

If you want to lose weight, you need to picture it. Start by lying down in a comfortable position, with your eyes closed, and distractions at a minimum. Then, begin to open yourself to possibility. Make sure that you understand what you want to see.

Work in stages. Firstly, visualize yourself standing in front of your mirror, day after day, looking thinner. You smile as you look in the mirror. You nod your head with positivity as you read the number on the scale. You have more lean muscle. Your face looks tighter. You have less thickness to your neck. Your fingers aren't as pudgy, your waist line is smaller; you feel lighter and fitter and your thighs are trimmer. Clothes seem looser.

Now, work your way back.

Begin to visualize things that are more specific. You already have the general, end-image of weight loss and satisfaction, now it's time to think smaller. Visualize yourself eating slowly at your table, on lunch at work, with family and friends, at a restaurant or place of residence. Visualize the smaller portions on the plate, the way they're so filling and healthy. Visualize an array of healthy foods, like fruits and vegetables, whole grains such as oatmeal, seafood and poultry, beans, nuts and seeds.

What matters most is not *what* you visualize eating, but *how* you visualize eating. Focus on eating mindfully, on enjoying every bite, on knowing that you are relishing food because it is nourishing, not because it drowns your sorrows, or forces you through a diet, or because you have to, or need to, or have no choice but *to*.

Eat because you *want* to. Because you want to take satisfaction in ingesting something that is delicious and nutritious. Don't imagine wolfing it down. Don't visualize yourself rushing through a meal. Make eating a healthy and enjoyable ritual of sorts. Savor the fact that you are eating smaller portions, and enjoying them more than bigger portions. The reason you enjoy them more is because you *know* that you are going to lose weight *and* be healthier.

Now move into another specific visualization. Perhaps you eat as a result of stress. Perhaps you eat out of boredom. Perhaps you simply eat as a reward for all your hard work. Or maybe you simply aren't getting the exercise you need and you know it. Whatever your honest appraisal of your situation, visualize it changing. Visualize waking up feeling refreshed and ready to go. Visualize yourself walking around your block, going to your gym, or taking small breaks in the middle of the day for yourself. Visualize yourself choosing water over soda, carrots over potato chips, fruit over ice-cream.

Amazingly, your brain will learn to see the world differently. This is where it all begins. Your brain will actually start to rewire itself. Your beliefs and perceptions will shift, so that pessimism and negativity give way to optimism and positivity.

They say that seeing is believing; but in reality, believing is seeing. If you cultivate the thought, the perception, it will literally manifest in everything you perceive. It will become engrained, an effortless part of your being that you no longer consciously activate. It will happen over hours and days and weeks, and as it strengthens, so too will your dedication to *the plan*.

Now that your neural networks are beginning to literally change their connections, it is time for the next step. It is time to start adding physical actions to your mental visualizations. Meditation and visualization are effective, but they are merely the stepping stone. To fully embrace weight loss and healthy living, you need to take action. You need to stick to *the plan*.

It doesn't have to be drastic, and it certainly won't happen overnight. But it *will* transform your life in the long-haul, in a way that is healthy, sustainable, and unbelievably uplifting.

So let's do it…

Shedding Your Insecurities

Diets don't matter.

That's right, let me say it again. Diets don't matter. Your *commitment* to them does.

So how strong is *your* commitment?

Too many times we rush to get something in our stomachs because our schedules are busy. "I need to grab a bite," we might think, and we rush off to the most convenient place for food on our lunch hours. Or maybe we pack a lunch, but we have so little time to eat, that when we do, we force it down. *Back to work, back to school, back to tasks and errands and my to-dos*, we think.

Gotta go, gotta go, gotta go. Time is of the essence

Or maybe we aren't in a rush, so what do we do? Well, we enjoy ourselves. We indulge. We relish the 'finer' things in life such as gratuitous portions and decadent desserts. We eat and eat, and appease our senses with an array of tasty, but unhealthy, choices and portions.

This is one of the problems with modern society. We don't make health a priority. And many times, it isn't entirely our fault. For many of us, good health insurance is harder to attain than ever before. For others, it's easy.

But even if it *is* easy, and we're well positioned, with a good job and nice benefits—are we living the way we should? Sure, we like to *think* we've got everything under control... But do we really?

"It's a good one," we might tell our friends and family and coworkers. "I save money. I get dental, vision, preventive, low monthly premiums—it's pretty comprehensive..."

And then what do we do? Well, if we're like most people, we rest on our laurels. Confident and secure in our health benefits, we worry about the doctor when it's time to visit or something comes up. Otherwise, we continue about our lives, unwilling to make the changes necessary to optimize our daily health.

And there always excuses.

I'm too tired

I'm too busy

I don't have enough money

I don't like exercising

Now's not a good time

I will tomorrow

I just can't lose weight

Diets don't work for me

Why bother?

What's the point?

Why is it all so hard?

So then what happens? Well, we go the easy route. We eat fast-food, we eat processed meals, we consume *what* we want *when* we want, or can, and then, on top of that, we don't exercise and we don't consider the consequences.

By and large, we consider other things more important. Working hard and making money is more important. Dealing with our kids, paying our bills, meeting coworkers, acquaintances, friends and family are more important.

Somehow, and for some reason, our own physical and mental wellbeing, the two facets of our lives that can literally improve *everything else*, become a second or third or fourth or fifth priority....

When we convince ourselves that we lack the time or resources to eat more healthy, we fail to recognize the truth: eating healthy is easy.

If you're too tired to make a healthy meal or to exercise, consider a simple fact: your body and brain are running on regular. What you want is *premium*.

When we eat healthier foods, we have more energy. We feel better. We think easier and spend less time doing things. We can work more efficiently, we can plan more effectively, we can think and act more rationally. So when you think that you don't have the energy to make a home-cooked meal, or don't have time to stick to a diet, think again.

Once you start the diet, you *will* have the time, energy, and resources to stick to it. Why? Because food is power! Fueling with the right stuff will ensure that you are ready to go. And the longer you stay at it, the easier it becomes!

Which brings us to the main question: *which diet is the best?*

Diets Don't Work, You Do: What You've Been Missing All Along

Remember what I said. No diet—that's *no diet*—is better than the other.

Scratching your head? Skeptical? Don't want to believe it? Well believe it.

Research shows that it doesn't really matter. It doesn't matter if you're doing the Atkins Diet, The Zone Diet, the Vegan Diet, the Vegetarian Diet, Weight Watchers, South Beach, Raw Food, Mediterranean—you name it. In fact, all of these diets have their reported benefits, just as all of them have their share of detractors and opponents.

Again, the main predictor of weight loss is sticking with the diet. That means not only following the specific protocol, but also maintaining that protocol for a lengthy period. The research doesn't lie. In numerous meta-analyses of the various diets, the only strong association found was between <u>diet adherence and resulting weight</u> <u>loss</u>. In other words, if a diet was effective, it was effective because a person stuck to it, not because of the actual protocols unique to the diet itself.

Problem is, diet adherence is no easy task. Although many people can lose weight for several months, most cannot maintain that weight loss. According to the National Health and Nutrition Examination Survey from 1999 to 2006, only 1 in 6 overweight and obese adults maintained weight loss of at least 10% for an entire year.

In a nutshell, worry less about the specific diet you're on, and more about just staying on it! There are no significant correlations between any one diet and weight loss. You can be eating raw foods all the time or tallying up points on weight watchers', and the weight loss you experience will be roughly the same (assuming you're consistent). Of course, if you're consistent with one and not another, you'll lose weight and become healthier on the one you're consistent with.

This may all sound good and well, but what does it actually mean? Does this mean that if all diets are about the same, there's no point in really having *any* diet? Do these findings basically invalidate the entire idea of dieting in the first place?

In short, the answer is no.

Of course, the real answer is a lot more complicated than that.

But before we get into those complexities, and the many competing theories of caloric intake, let's overview some basic steps to take. Whether keen on a particular diet, or simply hoping to improve general eating habits, here are a few things to consider…

Balance

In many ways, balance is the key to life. You want a balance of work and fun. A balance of stress and relaxation. You never want to do so much of one thing that it comes to dominate your living. If you find yourself totally engrossed in doing something or thinking something, you're missing out!

The same applies to eating. Experts everywhere may disagree over which foods ensure the quickest weight loss, but most of them do agree on one thing: eat a little bit of everything. The food pyramid is a little dated these days, but its general message holds true. You want to incorporate all the food groups into your diet.

So what does this mean exactly?

Easy: Before thinking about exact calorie intake, think about the source of those calories. Try to shoot for the rainbow. When you eat fruit, eat all the colors—blueberries, strawberries, grapes, oranges, limes, lemons, etc. Aim for a variety of vegetables too, including green ones and other colors like red potatoes, carrots and peppers. Focus especially on green vegetables such as kale, lettuce, spinach, collards, mustard greens, zucchini, asparagus, etc. The leafier your green vegetables, the more nutrient-dense. The more colorful your fruit medley, the more vitamin-dense.

When it comes to grains, think whole-grain. This means bread, brown rice, oatmeal, and the like. When it comes to meals, eat seafood like fish, oysters and clams. Eat poultry, eat eggs, and go for lean meats (they are marked at the grocery store by %). When it comes to dairy, don't be afraid to try different cheeses such as gouda, which has great anti-cancer properties. Also, experiment with soy milk or rice milk, anything with concentrated vitamin d and calcium values.

When eating in balance, remember to eat breakfast every day to prevent overeating later on. Choose fruit over fruit juice, and cut down on heavy olive oil use—no need to *drench* your vegetables in oil! Also, make it a rule of thumb to avoid sugar. Use water or juice cleanses to replace sugar-loaded fruit juices and soda. And always, make it a habit to avoid refined grains in white bread, rice, and pasta. These can lead to digestive issues among other health concerns.

This balanced approach to eating is good for many health problems, including diabetes, blood pressure, and energy levels, to name a few. Some will call this the DASH Diet, but more generally, it is just a healthy, invigorating plan for good eating and living. The beauty of eating in balance is that your body works in symbiosis. Some vegetables aid in the digestion of fats. Some legumes help certain meats to release their most nutritious contents. Certain fruits and grains activate each other in ways they would not if not eaten together.

Balance, balance, balance!

Frequency and Quality

Guess what? It's better to eat more often than less often. Sound good?

Well, there's a catch. What this doesn't mean is that you stuff your face whenever possible. What it *does* mean is that you eat smaller, healthier meals more often. The latest research indicates 5-6 meals a day, with each meal being smaller than if you were to shove down two or three a day. This is good because it keeps your metabolism chugging and doesn't stagnate you with oversized helpings. Your body is designed to receive constant small amounts of fuel. Throwing a ton of logs on the fire once or twice a day is much less efficient than feeding the flames smaller sticks throughout the day. Not to mention, all this constant small-sized eating will tempt you from binging or eating less healthy foods.

When it comes to snacking, it's important to choose delicious and nutritious alternatives to your typical pretzels, potato chips, and other vending machine temptations. Try low-fat or fat-free yogurt for starters. If you don't like yogurt, go for fresh, canned or dried fruit. Sliced vegetables such as carrots or celery stalks are good too. A great and easy snack/mini meal is a tomato sandwich. A grilled cheese with whole grain bread is also a solid choice.

When it comes to getting your day going, make sure your breakfast choices are smart. You want sustainable energy, not something that's going to spike you up and leave you crashing in no time. Consider fruit smoothies from frozen fruit and low-fat yogurt; cereals low in fiber and low in sugar like Total; and maybe some whole-wheat toast with a little bit of low-fat cheese. Top your oatmeal with fresh fruit and nuts, using low-fat or soy milk. All of these food choices are healthy, hearty, energy-providing options that will get your day off on the right foot.

If you're a morning coffee drinker, consider putting cinnamon in your Joe instead of sugar or sugar substitutes. If you're a butter and toast kind of person, consider trying the countless benefits of conut oil instead of butter. And definitely instead of margarine. Margarine can be chock full of funky chemicals that most people are unaware of.

Mindful Eating

What is mindful eating, you ask? Well, in a nutshell it's simply enjoying what you eat. Studies show that the brain takes 10 to 15 minutes to tell us that we're full. This means you can cram a lot of food in your mouth and gut before you're full. This explains why people will go all day without food, stuff themselves like pigs, and then feel almost nauseous. By the point the 10-15 minutes expires, all the food that was shoveled in is finally catching up with them.

So eat mindfully! Enjoy your healthy changes and the nutritious but delicious foods you've selected. Contrary to what many people think, healthy foods aren't bland or nasty. And feel free to reduce the size of your plate to potentially trick your brain into thinking you're eating more.

A Sustainable Plan

That's right, the key word is "sustainable." Natural weight loss is about more than simply losing weight. It's about keeping that weight *off*. It's about going through each and every new day with the confidence and *the plan* to stay motivated, stay fit, and stay the course. A realistic starting goal for most people is to shed 5-10 percent of your starting weight. This is both an attainable short-term goal, and a goal that will have immediate health benefits.

However, maybe your goals are more varied. Perhaps you want to do more than simply shave some percentage. Maybe you want to limit your intake of certain foods or beverages. Perhaps you want to incorporate a certain amount of exercise per week, or a certain amount of home-cooked meals. Maybe you have a guilty pleasure that you want to reduce to a consistent number…

Whatever your goal or goals, remember: (1) specificity; (2) attainability; and (3) imperfection. Don't shoot for the stars right off the bat if your feet are still firmly planted on the couch! Be realistic. You're not going to be able to run for

30 minutes 3 days a week if you've barely ever run in your life. You have to build up to it. And you're not going to be able to lose 5 pounds in a week or so (aside from water weight) unless you go on some kind of fasting. It's important to set goals that you can reach and that you can articulate. They should feature precise weight losses, numbers, or instances. And most importantly, they should be imperfect. You can't achieve the ideal right away. You'll have some struggles, and you have to mentally prepare yourself for those.

This is where all that visualization comes into place that we talked about earlier. Remember, visualization is still in play. You should be consistently visualizing the next incremental step, especially as you get into the thick of your plan.

But more about the plan.

See, when it comes to a plan, we have a couple of techniques in our pockets that we can use. One of them is the idea of gradual approximation. You don't jump immediately to 45% calorie reduction—and expect to sustain it. What you need to do is guide yourself, and allow your body to acclimate naturally. Start at 25%, after a week or so, work to 30%, then to 35% and so on. Work your way up step by step to that desired exercise time or frequency.

You *need* to be patient.

Get it in your brain that the key to success and longevity is commitment. And commitment, dear reader, requires an undeniable time investment. Remember, this is a lifestyle change, not simply a fad or brief diet. It's going to take a little bit of time.

But that's okay!

You might not like the idea of putting in effort over time, but effort is good (it burns calories). Not to mention, it's not as if you're simply forcing yourself through endless trials and tribulations. Enacting and sustaining a plan doesn't have to be hard. You'll get used to it, and it *will* become the norm.

Also, you can reward yourself.

Just be sure you aren't rewarding with more food. A lot of people like to have a 'cheat' day, but many times this sabotages the plan. You end up rewarding smaller and smaller accomplishments, to the point where you're basically cheating all the time.

Then you're back to square one.

So don't be a square-one person. When you reward yourself, do so with either a tangible thing, or something intangible. The reward should be meaningful and of a similar magnitude to your achievement. In other words, if you lose 10 pounds over a certain period, you would reward yourself with less than say if you achieve a greater goal of losing 25 or 30 lbs.

Rewards can be a fun experience at a ballgame, movie, theatre, party, festival, theme park, etc. They can also be items that you buy for yourself. If you opt for an intangible reward, consider something like a day to yourself, not worrying about errands or to-dos, or some other mind-pleasing, non-material activity.

Just be sure that you don't get caught up in dangerous associations. These associations will leave us stuck in bad habits that we are trying to erase. Such associations include eating in front of the T.V., grabbing an unhealthy snack during commercials, stopping for unhealthy food when we pass some place on the way to and from work, or pairing any number of activities with eating poorly.

If need be, you will have to change your daily routes and habits, if not just a little, to ensure that you don't fall slave to old habits. Again, apply visualization so that you're going strong. Visualize yourself opting for that healthy alternative when these old cues inevitably occur.

Self-Evaluation

This is another important part of eating and living healthily. Too many people get too down on themselves when they aren't losing weight as they expect. This is a problem. Don't expect to shred pounds immediately. Most diets that claim this are not going to sustain long-term. They're going to cut weight, usually too fast to be good for you, and then you're going to feel crappy. You'll be hungry, you'll be tired, and you'll hate yourself for feeling so.

So remember, *long-term*. When charting your progress, monitor it regularly. You can use a graphic display if you'd like, or you can just jot down weights. For the sake of your self-esteem, remember one thing: a single day's pattern of activity and diet *will not* have any real impact on your weight the following day. Your body's water weight will change from day to day, often due to things that have nothing to do with your plan.

And speaking of that plan, don't be dismayed when you get sidetracked. Seek the help of family and friends. Join message boards and online communities. Eat smaller meals at restaurants, and take home what you don't finish—don't feel pressured to eat it all at once. Stick to your shopping lists, and try to have meals at an actual table, instead in front of the T.V. or computer.

And best of all, keep a Food Log. This record or catalogue of your daily eating habits will keep you on the ball. You'll know why you feel the way you do, and how certain foods register in your mind and body. You'll also actively express your feelings, instead of bottling them up and giving up or giving in prematurely.

Take a look at the following Food Log as an example. Visualize how you could fill in the remaining blocks. Better yet, visualize how the foods and emotions/thoughts would become more healthy and positive as you progress in your plan.

Time	Food	Emotions/Thoughts	Ways to Improve
8:00 a.m.	Coffee and donut	Hungry but in a hurry	Orange juice, fruit, eggs
11:15 a.m.	Bagel Bites and Sprite	Really getting hungry	Carrots, sandwich, milk
4:30 p.m.	Wendy's chicken sandwich	Tastes good but feeling sluggish	
7:30 p.m.	....	....	....
10:45 p.m.	....	....	....

In the end, the Food Log is all about monitoring your behaviors and cognitions. You need to learn how to be self-evaluative without being self-deprecating. Appraise and admit your changing feelings. Know your shortcomings and chart how you're going to change your game. Don't be afraid to dig inside your head and really see what you're doing wrong.

And if you're wrong, you're wrong. That doesn't mean you're stupid, or forever fat, or incapable of following a diet and losing weight. What it *does* mean is that you're learning. You're becoming more informed and more capable. You're gaining in strength, in the ability to overcome obstacles that would have once derailed you.

But this isn't enough.

Because the equation is a little more complex than previously thought. And when it comes right down to it, there's a lot to be said on the topic of losing weight. Not just losing weight, but losing calories. And boosting your metabolism. And making the most of the diet (whichever it is) that you so choose….

The Calorie Conundrum – Are All pounds Created Equal?

Although research indicates that diets are only as successful as their consistency, many people beg to differ. And this should be no surprise. After all, there are a million diets for a million reasons. Some people want to eat more raw vegetables. Some people want to improve their heart health, or their brain power, or completely eliminate fat. Other people are anti-carbs, some people want to mix it all together, and certain eaters believe that nothing but marbled steaks is the path to eternal salivation and weight loss salvation.

Because most popular diets are based on their own frameworks of scientific evidence, there is never a shortage of reasons to give them a go. While the main predictor of weight loss is adherence, in certain cases, there just *might* be credence to one diet over another. That said, you have to be careful. Weight loss doesn't necessarily mean better health.

And sometimes, there's just not enough evidence to tell one way or the other.

Consider the unique case of the Twinkie Diet. That's right, the "Twinkie Diet." Never heard of it? Well, then prepare yourself. When a Professor Haub of human nutrition decided to go on a 10-week diet, he made a special commitment to himself: junk food would become his *main* food. Immediately, he began to eat twinkies and donuts, doritos, cookies and sugary cereals.

Of course, there was a catch. Haub believed that the nutritional content of his food would not matter, so long as he consumed less calories than he burned. Therefore, he consumed 1800 calories, 800 beneath the typical 2,600 daily consumption of a man his size.

As the diet progressed, his received the majority of his calories from junk food. But there *was* something healthy to his method. Every day, Haub made sure to take a multivitamin pill, drink a protein shake, and eat green vegetables such as beans or celery. By the end of his 10 week experiment, he had shed almost 30 pounds, his body fat dropped almost 10%, and his good and bad cholesterol levels had increased and decreased 20%, respectively. Despite everything he thought he knew about dieting, Haub's 'Twinkie Diet' seemed to be improving his weight and his health.

Of course, this is just one case for one man. Although Haub attributed the weight loss to portion control, what he couldn't explain was if he was truly healthier as a result. There was no telling what carcinogenic results could stem from his efforts—or what illnesses could arise if he sustained such a diet longer. Or better yet, if biological markers such as body fat, cholesterol and BMI are even accurate measures of health to begin with.

This is where things can get sticky. Most experts agree that if you're going to lose weight, you might as well opt for foods that are nutritious. While many people hop on fad diets that promise to shed weight no matter the food, these can be deceiving. Chances are, you've seen the documentary Supersize Me, about the man who eats nothing but McDonalds for 30 days straight. Although he could have theoretically eaten less calories every day and *lost* weight instead of gaining like he did, it's likely that he would have felt terrible doing so. This is because certain highly processed foods simply make us feel bad. They lower our energy levels, ruin our moods, and bring on bodily problems such as headaches, lethargy, fatigue, cramps, gastrointestinal issues, and potentially chronic diseases. They may enable weight *loss*, but the real question is: do they enable weight *maintenance*?

That is to say, are there certain diets that are better at keeping the pounds off once we've lost them? Diets that make us feel good and allow us to continue on the right track? Diets that are easier to adhere to than others, even if others may guarantee quicker but unsustainable results?

The research may surprise you…

Surprising Facts of a Faster Metabolism

As it turns out, a calorie is more than just, well, a calorie.

For anybody struggling with weight, this statement rings true. Sure, you can spend minute after minute, day after day, tracking the precise consumption of meals and calories, but what if you're still not losing weight? If your diet emphasizes quantity over all else, number over nutrition—think again.

What matters is more than simply the quantity of calories. In fact, research is beginning to show that the *quality* of calories consumed affects the *quantity* of calories consumed. Yes, it is true that taking in less calories than you burn will lead to weight loss. However, if those calories are coming from less-than-reputable sources, will they maintain that weight loss?

What we know about calories is that not all are created equal. When it comes to utilizing these units of energy, our bodies like to burn them in three ways. Firstly, we burn them just by staying alive. When you're sitting on the couch, in your car, at your desk, asleep in your bed. Resting takes energy. Especially if you're physically resting while your brain goes to work. But simpler than that, the basic processes of your organs require energy; consistent, measurable energy.

Secondly, our bodies burn calories in acts of physical exertion. This one is a no-brainer. When your heart rate's up and your lungs are on fire, your body is doing its thing. Walking, running, lifting weights, swimming, playing basketball or a game of Ping-Pong—all of these burn calories at a faster rate than resting. Using your muscles and your organs on a regular basis will ensure that calories are burning at an accelerated rate.

Finally, the third way our bodies burn calories is through waste. We lose heat through our extremities like our head, our fingers and toes. Heat loss is the result of 'thermogenesis, which is basically our bodies' attempts to stay warm. When you shiver, you're expressing thermogenesis. Ginger, guar gum, and caffeine and EGCG found in green tea are all promoters of thermogenesis.

Basically, the best way to lose weight and maintain it, is to consume good calories—and less of them. By introducing a gradual caloric restriction, we impose a semi-acute stress response that can actually extend our lives significantly. Not to mention, we feel better as a result.

But it *has* to be gradual. What most people fail to understand is that fast weight-loss diets go against human nature. These popular weight loss regimens trigger a starvation signal that will actually change our hormonal levels for the worse. This happens because our body has naturally built-in defense mechanisms. When weight is dropped too quickly, our brain tells our body to perceive food, all foods, as more appealing. This trigger means that we experience a variety of negative symptoms such as headaches, stomach problems, and weakness, in addition to a constant and growing craving for sustenance.

This is why the quality of our calories matter. A burger from Wendy's may have the same caloric content as a healthier alternative, but that healthier alternative more fully *satiates* our mind and body. In the end, the healthier alternative staves off our brain's starvation alert system, allowing us to more easily adapt to caloric restriction.

See, when it comes to caloric restriction and caloric quality control, what we need to understand is that all metabolisms are different. For some people, losing weight will never be easy. This is a phenomenon that scientists are just starting to understand, but the facts are emerging: your metabolism, especially if you've struggled with weight, may never reach a truly 'normal' level.

Consider a study at Columbia University wherein the metabolic systems of participants were closely scrutinized. Following a liquid diet that led to a 10% weight loss in all participants, the researchers collected data on participant weight *maintenance*. The results were surprising.

What they found was that the weight-reduced body has a different metabolism than a non-weight-reduced body of the same age and weight. In other words, those who dieted successfully and lost weight would have to consume fewer calories per day—as much as 300, 400, or 500 fewer—just to maintain their new weight. This seemed like an odd finding at first, but was quickly linked to very real physical changes within the body. It was discovered that muscle fibers became more slow-twitch in nature following weight loss, causing them to burn as much as 25% fewer calories during activity than those of a person naturally at that weight. This downturn in energy expenditure is disconcerting, to say the least.

Fortunately, there *are* ways to curb this problem. One promising study found that the best way to keep weight off following a loss of at least 10% is to seek a balance between *glycemic index* and *overall carbohydrate consumption*. The glycemic index (GI) is a measure of carbohydrates on a scale from 0 to 100 according to how much they raise blood sugar levels following consumption. Foods with a high GI are rapidly absorbed and digested and associated with drastic changes in blood-sugar levels; low-GI foods are slower and produce gradual rises in blood sugar and insulin levels. These foods delay hunger and have numerous benefits, especially in the fight against diabetes and heart disease.

According to the study, low-fat diets are not the way to go. These diets cause slower energy expenditure at both resting and during exercise. On the other hand, low-carbohydrate diets optimize energy expenditure and metabolic processes, *but* contribute to physiological stress and chronic inflammation. The third type of diet, the low-glycemic index diet, has smaller but similar positive benefits of the low-carb diet, but *does not* have any of the negative effects of stress or inflammation.

Put simply, the low-glycemic index diet is the best option for long-term weight loss and maintenance. In the aforementioned study, the participants consumed a low-glycemic diet comprised of 40% from carbohydrates, 40% from fat, and 20% from protein. If you're wondering the glycemic index of a given food, check here. And if you're wondering how much a 'normal person' of your weight should consume in terms of calories, check here.

And if you're now more confused than ever, and feel like it's all too much work just to keep off some stupid pounds, keep reading...

Sleep, Exercise and Fat-Burning Foods—What You NEED to Know

You might be pretty tired of it all at this point.

Glycemic index? Carb values? Metabolic changes and starvation signals?? All I want is to lose some $^&@ weight!

Well don't fret. You're learning what it takes and if you've come this far, you can't stop now. Your life will improve as a result. Besides, it's not *all* difficult. Believe it or not, there are actually some easy steps you can take to start losing weight. If you crave more concrete steps for shedding pounds, check these:

Exercise

Yea, yea, you've heard this one before. Maybe you've heard it so many times, that the thought of getting up and getting moving is practically nauseating. Even if it is, you need to hear it again. <u>NASA studies</u> show that just a couple of days of inactivity can stall our metabolism, and even permanently change it. Fortunately, if you get moving a little every day, you *will* accelerate your metabolism.

But it's more than that.

Exercise that builds muscle mass is the best. While it's true that aerobic exercise is wonderful for killing calories, strength training is the key to big metabolic changes. Functional fitness activities that feature kettle bells, hand weights and stretch bands are great ways to build up your triceps, biceps, abs and burn away fat. If you don't like the thought of all this strength stuff, consider doing it in your downtime. When you're watching television or a movie, or waiting to do something else, do some repetitions, lift some weights—and get *ripped*!

Be warned, however: exercise is not as effective as dieting. That is to say, exercising alone will not result in more weight loss than dieting alone. Especially in <u>overweight or obese post-menopausal women.</u>

Think about it. Attaining the same benefits through exercise can be trying. Sometimes it would take you a good 40 minutes of aerobic exercise to get the same benefits as foregoing an unhealthy snack like Doritos. When relying on only exercise, we have a tendency to overcompensate. We get hungrier and our hormones start acting up. Many times, we negate our good exercise by then 'cheating' afterwards with a bucket of fried chicken and some beer (or something to the like).

Not to mention, rigorous exercise can actually be a detriment. If you bust your butt in a morning workout and spend the rest of the day too exhausted to do *anything*, you might actually end the day having burned less calories than if you had never done that workout at all.

Again, your best bet is to combine exercise with dieting. This may sound like a tall-order, but it becomes much easier once you realize how delicious healthy foods can taste.

Sleep

Obviously we all need sleep. But if you're getting up early and hoping that your morning coffee-to-go will suppress your appetite and make up for lost Zsss, *think again.* In fact, getting lots of sleep is a great way to keep you thinner. The body is actually most metabolically varied during sleep, so the longer we're asleep, the more we churn the engine—you burn more fat at a lower energy level.

If you start missing too much sleep, you will also begin to mess with important hormones, ghrelin and leptin, which deal with hunger and feelings of satiation. In other words, if you are routinely sleep-deprived, your brain will signal to your body that you need food all the time. Worse yet, you will be unable to feel satiated, and will continue to crave foods that have cheap but high energy investments (such as sugary snacks).

Hormonal Imbalance

One of the main sources of hormonal imbalance is hypothyroidism. Hypothyroidism is a condition in which the pituitary gland produces inadequate amounts of a hormone that regulates metabolism. This can lead to exhausting weight gain that may resist your best diet and exercise efforts. 20% of adults over 40 have an underactive thyroid. When considering if you need to have a thyroid test, consider the symptoms: fatigue and lethargy, feelings of coldness, poor circulation in extremities, hair loss (even of eyebrows and eyelashes) and an unchangeable weight gain that does not respond to your strongest efforts.

Don't be afraid to get tested!

And Finally....

Fat-Burning Foods

Yes, there *are* foods that will help you burn fat faster than you probably realized. They are:

Pine Nuts

Remember that hormone ghrelin that is critical during sleep? Well, pine nuts just so happen to boost its levels, meaning that enough nuts will get you feeling nice and full. Pine nuts and almonds are practically interchangeable. Both will also help cut down on belly fat.

Eggs

Forget all the health hazards you've heard concerning eggs. In fact, these delicious little morsels are great for your health. As a concentrated form of animal protein, eggs supply a lot of energy and don't carry that extra fat you get from meats. Throw in an egg with your toast, coffee, and cereal, and you've got one *heck* of a start to your day.

Oats

These whole grains are rich in soluble fiber and will

reduce your blood fat and cholesterol. They also make you feel very full and will help you ease into sleep.

Apples

An apple or two a day keeps the doctor at bay—and the pounds. Because of their pectin content, apples reduce the amount of fact your body can absorb, and also fill you up with their fiber content. Consistent apple-eating can also help prevent high cholesterol, high blood pressure, and prediabetes that leads to a thick waist.

Great for a late night snack!

Cinnamon

This little spice has a million and one benefits. Well, not a million, but plenty of enough to give you pause. So add a little spice in your day. Cinnamon is one of life's <u>premiere health hacks.</u>

<u>Alrighty</u>

By this point your head is probably swimming. We've gone over some interesting studies, we've explored the latest research on foods and calories, we've even shed some light on the deep physical and psychological processes involved in dieting and exercise.

If you're confused and don't know where to go from here, start simple. Remember, visualize first and visualize always, and slowly choose the diet that you can truly envision working. Except, don't consider it a diet, per se. Remember, this is a <u>lifestyle</u> change.

But it's okay if you don't want that. If you're rather pop a pill, have surgery, or try some fast weight-loss fad, by all means go ahead. At the end of the day, it's your body and your mind and your choice where to go in life. What may work for you may not for others; what works for others may fail every time for you.

No matter what road or cookbook you decide to take, keep in mind the end prize. I argue that it's better to go naturally than it is to destroy your body long-term for short-term gains. Of course, that all depends on your goal. Many people in society find that life is about the present. Plenty of people forfeit their futures to live wild and crazy in the present.

If you want to go wild and crazy, seeking nothing more than a hot trimmer body a couple weeks from now—then go for it. After all, the future is never guaranteed.

Besides, I'm not here to cast value judgments. But hopefully, sincerely, you'll find something from this book that helps you.

After all, the point of reading this book is to achieve weight loss and weight maintenance *for life*. So best of luck in your journey.

Sincerely,

C.K. Murray

A Special Note:

Thank you for reading "*Natural Weight Loss: PROVEN Strategies for Healthy Weight Loss & Accelerated Metabolism.*" If you enjoyed reading this book and would like to be included on an email list for when similar content is available, feel free:

Sign-Up Now

As always, thank you for reading.

And may you continue to live healthily and happily.

Sincerely,

C.K. Murray

Other works by C.K. Murray: